*To care for those who once cared for us is one of the Highest Honors*

-Tia Walker

# Disclaimer

This handbook is published for guidance and brief summaries of information for; caregivers, family members and/or advisors. While our best efforts have been used in preparing this handbook, we strongly advise you to always consult your local professionals and resources. Therefore, neither the authors nor the publisher shall be held liable or responsible to any person or entity with respect to any loss or incidental or consequential damage caused, or alleged to have been caused, directly or indirectly, by the information contained herein. Authors are not part of any government agency or affiliated with one.



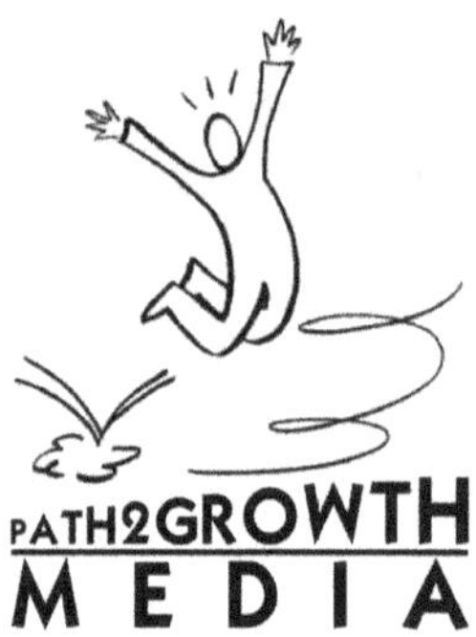

ISBN 978-0-9974865-0-6
Path2Growth Media
Beach Haven, NJ 08008
www.LorraineSpiotta.com

# Key Solutions for Caregivers
## Unlock for the answers...



Lorraine Kenney Spiotta, CLU, ChFC
and
Tracey Christenson Wolfman, RN, BSN, MA


Edited by Susanne Whited

# Authors' Note

The process of step-by-step and day-to-day caregiving for a family member or some loved one is not an easy task - it is complex, sometimes stressful, and it must be approached seriously and thoroughly.

This handbook has been researched and written with the thought that it might inspire you to make an effort to understand and learn how to prepare and organize yourself to meet such a challenge head-on. In addition, we are hopeful it will provide you with some helpful guidance and advice as you proceed through the process.

As a caregiver, you should know that you are not alone in having this kind of experience; countless others have encountered just such a situation. The informative material contained in the following pages will be of value to you and your care-giving experience will be much easier.

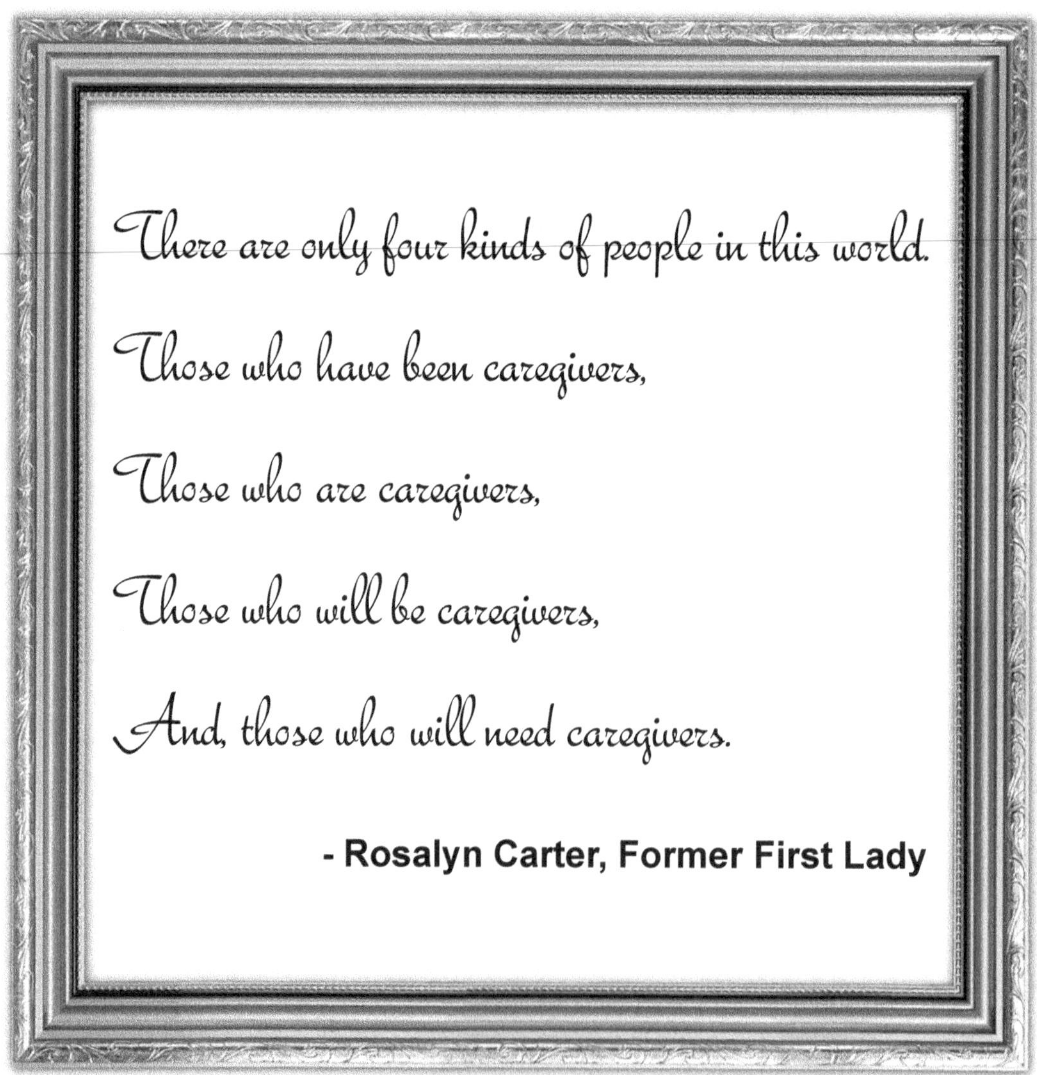

# Table of Contents

# Keep your information up to date!

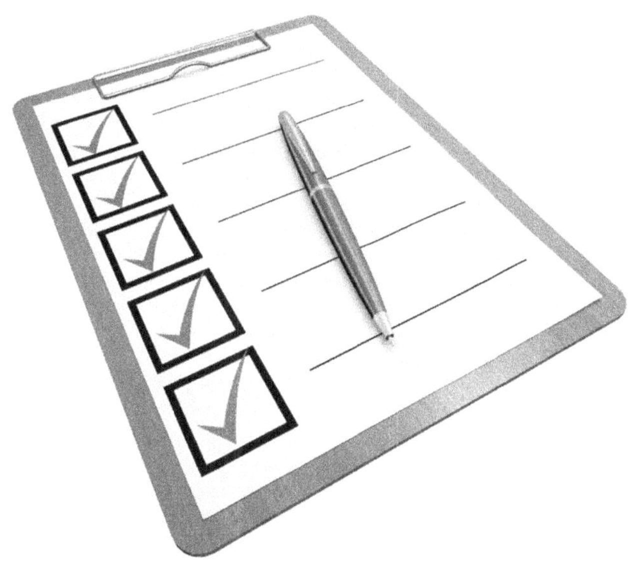

Go to

**KeySolutionsForCaregivers.com**

and get your

# FREE

printable copy

of the forms in this book!

## Your Packet Includes These Worksheets:

Personal Information

Financial Information

Primary Doctor Information

Health Assessment Report

Daily Medication Schedule

Master List of Medications

Specialists Information

Most Recent Hospitalizations

List of Questions for Care Recipient's Doctor

Cost of Care

What's Your Plan

Exploring Long Term Care Insurance

## KeySolutionsForCaregivers.com

# Section I

Personal Information

Financial Information

Primary Doctor Information

Health Assessment Report

Daily Medication Schedule

Master List of Medications

Specialists Information

Most Recent Hospitalizations

List of Questions for Care Recipient's Doctor

**Personal information, legal documents, list of assets, list of medications, and login and passwords will need to be accessible for the caregiver. However, because this information is private, keep it somewhere safe.**

Hospitals and doctors will need a copy of a current Advanced Directive/Living Will and medication list. Having a list of bank accounts and other assets will be important for federal, state, county and/or veteran benefits. Documents such as marriage and divorce decrees may also be necessary. Check with your local Office on Aging for grant programs and eligibility requirements.

Don't forget to update information if and when it changes in any way.

**Name**: ________________________________________________

Date of birth : ________________________  Social security number: ________________

Health insurance carrier: ______________  ID#: ________________________

Phone number: ________________________  Date of birth of spouse: ______________

**Attorney name**: ________________________________________

Attorney phone: ________________________________________

Documents needed:
- **Advanced directive/living will** outlines recipient's wishes in regard to staying on life support or not. Two physicians and/or specialist must determine life expectancy.
- **Health care proxy** which authorizes designated person to discuss with physicians the medical treatment for the care recipient who is unable to communicate his/her wishes.
- **Financial power of attorney** gives designated person authority to transact affairs of care recipient while he/she is alive.
- **Will** is for the distribution of assets at time of passing.
- **Birth certificate/marriage certificate/divorce decree** may be needed for Veteran benefits and/or other benefits.

Burial plot or other arrangements: ________________________________

Cemetery information: ________________________________________

Funeral home: ________________________________________________

Special Instructions: ________________________________________

**Medicare has four parts: Parts A and B (referred to as 'Original' or 'Basic' Medicare) are provided by the federal government. What is sometimes referred to as Part C and Part D are provided by private insurance carriers and supplement the coverage in Original Medicare by providing additional or increased benefits.**

Medicare Part A -  Qualification information provided in section II.

Medicare Part B                                                 current premium: _______

Medicare Advantage Part C                          current premium: _______

Medicare Part D - prescription drug insurance coverage.          current premium: _______

Medicare Supplement: _________ plan letter: _________ current premium: _______


## Military Records

Military identification number: ______________________________

Eligible for veteran benefits: ______________________________

Location of nearest veteran skilled nursing facility: ______________

Contact information: ________________ Cost of care: ____________

Other benefits available: ______________________________


## Long Term Care Insurance

Insurance company: ______________________________

Policy number: ______________________________

Phone number: ______________________________

Insurance agent: ______________________________

Phone: ________________ Email: ________________

## Life Insurance Policies

Insurance company:

Policy number:

Amount of death benefit:                    Cash value:

Beneficiary:


Insurance company:

Policy number:

Amount of death benefit:                    Cash value:

Beneficiary:


Insurance company:

Policy number:

Amount of death benefit:                    Cash value:

Beneficiary:


## Banking Information (Login and passwords should be kept somewhere safe.)

Name of Bank:                    Branch location:

Account number:                    Type of account:


Name of Bank:                    Branch location:

Account number:                    Type of account:

Name of Bank: ____________________   Branch location: ____________________

Account number: ____________________   Type of account: ____________________


Name of Bank: ____________________   Branch location: ____________________

Account number: ____________________   Type of account: ____________________


**Investment Accounts** (Login and passwords should be kept somewhere safe.)

Financial planner/stock broker: ____________________

Name: ____________________

Phone: ____________________   Email: ____________________


Name of financial company: ____________________   Branch: ____________________

Type of account: ____________________   Account number: ____________________

Website: ____________________   Telephone number: ____________________

Other: ____________________


Name of financial company: ____________________   Branch: ____________________

Type of account: ____________________   Account number: ____________________

Website: ____________________   Telephone number: ____________________

Other: ____________________


Name of financial company: ____________________   Branch: ____________________

Type of account: ____________________   Account number: ____________________

Website: _______________________    Telephone number: _______________________

Other: _______________________________________________________________

Name of financial company: _______________    Branch: _______________________

Type of account: _______________________    Account number: _______________________

Website: _______________________    Telephone number: _______________________

Other: _______________________________________________________________

Name of financial company: _______________    Branch: _______________________

Type of account: _______________________    Account number: _______________________

Website: _______________________    Telephone number: _______________________

Other: _______________________________________________________________

Name of financial company: _______________    Branch: _______________________

Type of account: _______________________    Account number: _______________________

Website: _______________________    Telephone number: _______________________

Other: _______________________________________________________________

Name of financial company: _______________    Branch: _______________________

Type of account: _______________________    Account number: _______________________

Website: _______________________    Telephone number: _______________________

Other: _______________________________________________________________

## Pension Information

Contact information:

Phone:

## Debt

Mortgage:

Car loan:

Other:

Other:

Other:

## Other Relevant Financial Information

**Coordinating care between doctors, specialists and inpatient hospital care is important and the more information you can provide, the more you will help streamline the process.**

Primary care/concierge physician

Name:

Phone:                                    Fax:

Address:

Which hospital does he/she have privileges with?

Date/reason for last visit:

Date/reason for last visit:

Date/reason for last visit:

Date:                          Prescribe medication for:

Date:                          Prescribe medication for:

Date:                          Prescribe medication for:

List ALL diagnosis and surgeries: i.e.; cancer, heart surgery, vascular disease, high blood pressure, back operation, removal of gallbladder etc…

Notes for next office visit:

**Record health assessment information as often as possible so you are prepared to get the best advice during the physician's appointment.**

Date: _______________________________________________________________

Blood Pressure:          standing _______ / _______     sitting _______ / _______

Reaction to medication: _______________________________________________

Constipation: _________________________________________________________

Light headed: _________________________________________________________

Up at night: __________________________________________________________

Tremors: _____________________________________________________________

Rash: ________________________________________________________________

| | | | |
|---|---|---|---|
| Breathing: | normal | some shortness | difficult |
| Speech: | normal | slurred | difficult |
| Awareness: | normal | occasionally confused | very confused |
| Memory Loss: | short term | long term | |
| Balance: | good | poor | |

## Need help?

| | | | |
|---|---|---|---|
| Getting out of bed/chair: | yes | sometimes | no |
| Standing: | yes | sometimes | no |
| Toileting: | yes | sometimes | no |
| Bathing: | yes | sometimes | no |
| Eating: | yes | sometimes | no |
| Dressing: | yes | sometimes | no |

**Other observations:** ___________________________________________________

_____________________________________________________________________

_____________________________________________________________________

**Daily Medication Schedule:** Keep updated and (2) copies with you. Be sure to include vitamins, herbal supplements and over the counter medication.

Allergies to medication: _______________________________________________

Allergies to food: ____________________________________________________

Pharmacy name/location: ______________________________________________

Phone: _______________________________     Fax: _______________________

## Morning

| Time | Medication | Dosage | Used for | Taken with food |
|------|-----------|--------|----------|-----------------|
|      |           |        |          |                 |
|      |           |        |          |                 |

## Afternoon

| Time | Medication | Dosage | Used for | Taken with food |
|------|-----------|--------|----------|-----------------|
|      |           |        |          |                 |
|      |           |        |          |                 |

## Evening

| Time | Medication | Dosage | Used for | Taken with food |
|------|-----------|--------|----------|-----------------|
|      |           |        |          |                 |
|      |           |        |          |                 |

## Notes and special instructions

**Master List of Medications: Be sure to include vitamins, herbal supplements and over the counter medication.**

Allergies to medication: ______________________________________________

Allergies to food: ___________________________________________________

Pharmacy name/location: ______________________________________________

Phone: _______________________________ Fax: _______________________

| Medication Name | Dosage | Time | How taken: i.e mouth, patch, injection |
|---|---|---|---|
|  |  |  |  |
|  |  |  |  |
|  |  |  |  |
|  |  |  |  |
|  |  |  |  |
|  |  |  |  |
|  |  |  |  |
|  |  |  |  |
|  |  |  |  |
|  |  |  |  |
|  |  |  |  |
|  |  |  |  |
|  |  |  |  |

**When a specific diagnosis has been determined, research locally for specialists, support groups and community resources.**

Specialty: _______________________     Doctor name: _______________________

Address: _______________________________________________________________

Phone number: _______________________     Fax number: _______________________

Diagnosis: _______________________     Medication prescribed: _______________________

Results/follow up: _______________________________________________________________

_______________________________________________________________________________

---

Specialty: _______________________     Doctor name: _______________________

Address: _______________________________________________________________

Phone number: _______________________     Fax number: _______________________

Diagnosis: _______________________     Medication prescribed: _______________________

Results/follow up: _______________________________________________________________

_______________________________________________________________________________

---

Specialty: _______________________     Doctor name: _______________________

Address: _______________________________________________________________

Phone number: _______________________     Fax number: _______________________

Diagnosis: _______________________     Medication prescribed: _______________________

Results/follow up: _______________________________________________________________

Admittance into the hospital is usually through the emergency room and possibly for a condition that is new and/or an accident has occurred. Knowing which hospital, the insured prefers and if the primary care physician has privileges is important. Also, be sure to take a current copy of the medication list and advanced directive/living will.  If moved to a rehabilitation facility, be sure to record that information as well.

Date admitted to hospital: _______________________  Date released: _______________

Reason: ______________________________________________________________________

Procedure and tests performed: _________________________________________________

Results/notes: ________________________________________________________________

____________________________________________________________________________

____________________________________________________________________________

Date admitted to hospital: _______________________  Date released: _______________

Reason: ______________________________________________________________________

Procedure and tests performed: _________________________________________________

Results/notes: ________________________________________________________________

____________________________________________________________________________

____________________________________________________________________________

Date admitted to hospital: _______________________  Date released: _______________

Reason: ______________________________________________________________________

Procedure and tests performed: _________________________________________________

Results/notes: ________________________________________________________________

____________________________________________________________________________

Write down any questions that should be asked of your doctors as they come up and be sure to take the list to doctor's appointments so the questions are not forgotten.

1.

2.

3.

4.

# Section II

Medicare

Medicare Part A

Medicare Part B

Medicare Part C

Medicare Supplement

Medicare Part D

**Medicare: The federally provided health insurance program that insures more than 40 million people - most over the age of 65.**

**What Medicare is - and isn't.**
Medicare has four parts. Parts A and B (referred to as 'Original' or 'Basic' Medicare) are provided by the federal government. What is sometimes referred to as Part C and Part D are provided by private insurance carriers and supplement the coverage in Original Medicare by providing additional or increased benefits.

**Important points to know.**
- Medicare is *not* free; you have to pay deductibles, premiums, co-pays.
- Medicare may *not* cover your dependents or spouse.
- Your employer will *NOT* notify or enroll you; it's up to you to know when to enroll.
- In most cases, Medicare will *not* notify you when it's time to enroll.
- Each Medicare Part has its own enrollment period and late enrollment penalty.
- Medicare does *not* cover every medical expense.
- Medicare may *not* cover you outside the United States.
- An *active* (current) employee enrolled in a group health plan is not required to enroll in Part 'B'.
- Enrolled in COBRA or a former employer's health plan is *not* considered being in an 'active employee's' health plan.

**Except in limited circumstances, 'Original' Medicare does *not* cover:**
- Private duty nursing
- Private room, television, telephone
- Vision, hearing and dental care
- Long term care in a nursing home
- Medical services provided outside the United States
- Most routine physical exams (Annual wellness checkups are covered.).

**Enrollment**
Each Medicare "Part" has its own enrollment period, late enrollment penalty, deductibles and premiums.

If you are already receiving Social Security benefits you will most likely automatically be enrolled in Medicare Parts A and B. **If not, you must enroll by contacting Medicare.**

## Medicare Eligibility - if older than age 65 (the normal age for receiving Medicare)

- You are a US citizen or have a resident visa.

- You qualify under your spouse's or former spouse's work record and he/she is at least 62.

and:

- You've been married for at least 1 year; or

- you *were* married for at least ten years and you haven't remarried before age 60.

## Medicare Eligibility - if younger than age 65 (and meet certain other requirements)

- You are receiving Social Security and Disability benefits for at least 24 months.

- You have permanent kidney failure (End Stage Renal Disease) or ALS.

## Part 'A' - Hospitalization Coverage

This part of the 'basic' insurance provides for coverage in a hospital or, in some cases, skilled nursing facility (SNF), and includes:

- Semi-private room

- All meals provided directly by the hospital or nursing facility

- The services of a professional nursing staff

- Other services provided by the hospital or nursing facility such as lab tests, medical appliances, rehabilitation services.

## Part A - Enrollment  (Initial Enrollment at age 65)

You must enroll during the 7-month period that:

- Begins 3 months before the month you turn 65

- The month you turn 65

- Ends 3 months after the month you turn 65.

Coverage begins on the first of your birth month.

## Who Pays for Part A?

If you have 40 or more 'credits' of Medicare-covered employment (ten years) Part A is 'premium free'. If you are not otherwise eligible for 'premium free' Part A, contact Medicare to determine your premium.

## Part A - Benefit Period Deductible

The Benefit Period:

- Begins the day you go into a hospital or skilled nursing facility (SNF);
- Ends when you haven't received any hospital or SNF skilled care for 60 consecutive days.
- If admitted into a hospital or a SNF after one benefit period has ended, a new benefit period begins.

Contact Medicare to determine the deductible amount which changes annually. Remember, this deductible period is NOT an annual deductible. For each benefit period you pay a 'co-pay' until day 150 at which point you pay the full cost of hospitalization.

## Part A includes Skilled Nursing Facility care with its own set of rules.

To be eligible for Medicare coverage in a Skilled Nursing Facility (referred to as SNF) you must have been in the hospital as a 'formally admitted patient', not 'under observation' for at least three days, not including the day of discharge, and the SNF must be Medicare approved.

Original Medicare covers stays in a SNF for up to 100 days in a benefit period with the first 20 days paid at 100% by Medicare. From day 21 to 100 you pay a co-pay.

Part A also provides coverage for **home health aides, durable medical supplies, medical social services** and **hospice care** with strict qualifying rules. Contact Medicare for specific rules.

**IMPORTANT:** The benefits described for Part A may be supplemented by additional coverage such as Medicare Advantage or Medicare Supplement ("Gap") insurance.

## Part 'B' - Medical

This part provides for doctors' services, certain outpatient services such as lab tests and certain drugs administered in a doctor's office.

## Part B does NOT cover:

- Long-term care
- Routine dental care
- Dentures
- Cosmetic surgery
- Acupuncture
- Hearing aids and exams for fitting hearing aids
- Other - check Medicare.gov.

Everyone enrolled in Part B pays a monthly premium, unless they're eligible for state assistance. This premium, like other Medicare charges such as deductibles and co-pays is subject to annual adjustments. If your income is more than a certain level, you pay more.


## Part B - Enrollment

If you have group health insurance from an employer as an 'active' employee check with your plan administrator to see if you are required to enroll in Part 'B' at age 65.

You may sign up within 8 months of your employer coverage ending under a 'Special Enrollment Period'. Enrolled in a retiree plan or COBRA does not constitute enrollment in a plan for 'active' employees.


## Part B - Late Enrollment

- There is a penalty for not signing up when first eligible.

- The penalty is 10% for each full 12-month period for as long as you have Part B.

- You sign up during a Special Enrollment Period. No penalty if you sign up within 8 months of employment or employer coverage ending.


## If you want additional or more coverage

There are two options if you want coverage beyond what 'Original Medicare' offers. Both are offered by private insurance carriers. Not all plans are available in all areas. Premiums may vary widely.


## Medicare Advantage

- Often referred to as Part C.

- Must enroll in Parts A and B.

- Choose PP, PFFS, HMO plan versions.

- Must go to Network provider in the service area.

- Out-of-pocket expenses limits determined by insurer.

- Annual limits you pay set by insurer.

- May include prescription, dental, vision.

- Can change plans only during annual open enrollment.

- Do not buy based on premium; read the small print.

## Medicare Supplement

- You must be enrolled in Parts A and B to purchase Medigap.

- Use any provider that accepts Medicare.

- Premiums may be higher than MA plans but usually have fewer out-of-pocket costs.

- Does not cover prescription drugs.

- Choice of several plan options. All Medigap plans with the same letter provide the same coverage.

## Part 'D' - Prescription Drug Coverage

Unless covered by some Medicare Advantage plans:

- Covers major portion of prescription drug costs

- You choose plan design and private insurance carrier

- Apply at age 65 or

- During annual open enrollment (Mid October - Early December) or special enrollment period for a January 1 start

- You may need proof of prior 'creditable prescription coverage'.

## What You Pay

All stand-alone Part D plans charge a monthly premium with varying fees. In addition you are responsible for paying an annual deductible and a co-payment for each prescription.

Depending on the cost of the drugs you use, you may move through 4 phases of coverage each calendar year.

- **Annual Deductible** - the amount you pay each year before insurance begins.

- **Initial Coverage Period** - You pay the required copays until the total cost of your drugs – what you and your plan have paid – reaches a certain amount from the beginning of the year.

- **Coverage Gap (The Donut Hole)** - Once your drug costs exceed the Initial Coverage limit, your plan pays nothing. (You may get a discount on brand-name drugs from the manufacturer or a discount on generic drugs from the government.)

- **Catastrophic Coverage** - Coverage resumes once you've met the limits in the 'donut hole' - Process begins again each January 1.

---

**To enroll in Medicare or for more Medicare information, go to Medicare.gov or call (800) 633-4227.**

---

# Section III

Medicaid

**Medicaid is designed to help people in need of financial assistance (aid) for medical and/ or long term care expenses. Each state administers its own Medicaid program - which means the rules and benefits often vary from state to state.**

The monthly cost of privately paying for a nursing home, can quickly deplete financial resources. Therefore, after paying for services on your own and/or relying on family and friends, the time may come to learn about Medicaid. Medicaid is a joint federal and state program providing free or low-cost health coverage for more than fifty million limited-income people.

Some important things to know:

- You may qualify for Medicaid based on your annual income. To do so, you must know the 'poverty level' for the current year. This will determine your eligibility.

- However, if your annual income is higher, a provision referred to as; "medically needed" may apply. Contact your state Medicaid program for specific details.

- Apply through your local Medicaid agency or www.healthcare.gov.

- Go to www.naela.org for a list of attorneys who practice Elder Law within your state.

- The Community Spouse Resource Allowance (CSRA) protects the spouse of the Medicaid applicant by allowing a certain amount of the couple's resources (money and other assets) to be retained for him/her to remain at home and within the community.

- Medicaid requires a list of all assets, "Resource Amount", a person owned or transferred within the past five years (60-months) from the date of the Medicaid application. This is referred to as the "Look-Back Period".

- Any gifts or transfers made within the past 60-months from the date of the application create a "penalty period".

- Each state determines its own average "Private Pay" cost of a nursing home called a "Penalty Divisor" and divides the dollar amount of the transfer by the average private pay divisor which will create a specific number of months where the person is penalized before Medicaid will pay for the nursing home stay.

For Example:

If one state's penalty divisor is $5,000 and another state's penalty divisor is $12,000 per month, a $10,000 gift would cause a two-month penalty period in the first state, but less than a one-month penalty period in the second.

Therefore, if the applicant wrote a check to his/her daughter for $10,000 and applied for Medicaid within five years from the date on the check, the state Medicaid office will use their average private pay cost of a nursing home of $5,000 and use this penalty divisor number to determine how many months the applicant must wait before Medicaid will pay for the nursing home.

> Gift to daughter is $10,000 / $5,000 (average private pay) = 2-month penalty period

> Or, the gift is $120,000 / $12,000 (average private pay) = 10-month penalty period

**Benefits**

States establish and administer their own Medicaid programs and determine the type, amount, duration, and scope of services within broad federal guidelines. States are required to cover certain "mandatory benefits," and can choose to provide other "optional benefits" through the Medicaid program.

Here is a list of mandatory (required) benefits that all state Medicaid programs must offer:

- Inpatient hospital services
- Outpatient hospital services
- EPSDT: early and periodic screening, diagnostic, and treatment services
- Nursing facility services
- Home health services
- Physician services
- Rural health clinic services
- Federally qualified health center services
- Laboratory and X-ray services
- Family planning services
- Nurse Midwife services
- Transportation to medical care
- Freestanding birth center services (when licensed or otherwise recognized by the state)
- Certified pediatric and family nurse practitioner services
- Tobacco cessation counseling for pregnant women

# Section IV

Physicians Who Make House Calls

Medication Management

Nutrition and Meals

Bathing

Personal Hygiene

Bathroom Assistance

Medical Supplies and Equipment

The pages that follow contain useful information on how best to handle the many functions you will encounter in your role as a caregiver. Caregiver Support Groups are of tremendous value to the caregiver. Support groups allow the person to express their feelings, share stories, get helpful information from others and know they are not alone. Many hospitals and organizations hold free caregiver support meetings regularly. Newspapers frequently print weekly and monthly support group meetings or you can contact your local hospital so that they may refer you to a local chapter.

## Physicians Who Make House Calls

The American Academy of Home Care Medicine can assist in locating physicians who make house calls and their website is www.aahcm.org. Home-care physicians can provide:

- Complete evaluations

- Wound care

- Blood work

- Prescribe medication

- EKG (electrocardiograms)

- May not be affiliated with hospital

## Medication Management

Administering medication can present a real challenge to some caregivers. Because some medications have an unpleasant taste, the person may refuse or just keep it in their mouth before discarding it later. Try to make sure the person is swallowing the medication (pills) and, if necessary, disguise it in food if they refuse or spit it out. If problem persists, speak to the physician or ask the pharmacist if liquid form is available.

- Always keep a current list of medications, including over-the-counter ones.

- Keep medication schedule and list of any allergies.

- To avoid dosing mistakes, set up pill boxes once a week.

- Keep applesauce and pudding on hand – mix pills with these if necessary.

- Pill-slicer or crusher is available at pharmacy.

- Set alarm reminders. Cells phones allow you set up the alarm times once and they will repeat the same time every day.

**Nutrition and Meals**

Make meal time a social time. The care recipient should sit in a comfortable position and continue to sit up for at least 20 minutes after eating. In order to promote independence, he/she should be encouraged to do as much as they can on their own.

- A balanced diet is important – high protein drinks, carbohydrates, fats, fruits and vegetables. Fluids are essential for hydration.

- Prior to sitting at the table, ascertain possible need to go to bathroom.

- Always encourage independence at meal time. Position plate for ease, provide flavorful food and handicap utensils.

- Bites of food should be alternated with sips of liquid (flexible straw is helpful) and small portions are more appealing.

- If necessary, you can butter bread, pour coffee/tea and cut meats.

- Notify physician if poor appetite is apparent.

- Look for signs of poor nutrition: weakness, sweating, sunken cheeks, diarrhea bouts, dry and reddened eyes, swollen and red patchy tongue, weight loss, trembling and poor muscle tone.

**Home Delivered Meals**: Local community based volunteer organizations throughout the country provide meals to the elderly homebound. These meals provide a nutritionally balanced meal usually once a day. Contact your local town for information. Catholic Charities and the United Way are organizations that also can assist with this.

Personal hygiene needs to be done on a daily basis, try to make things as simple as possible. Sponge bath or shower improves circulation and provides a sense of well-being. Sometimes, due to limitations or illness, it can become a challenging task that will be met with great resistance.

**Bathing**

- Determine if person prefers a bath or a shower - try to maintain the same routine. Shower benches or chairs are helpful and available through a medical supply company.

- Gather all supplies before bringing the person into the shower (keep a check list for repeated use).

- For reasons of safety, provide grab rails for holding on inside and outside of the shower.

- Hand-held shower heads work best - have non-slip mats on the floor.

- Keep person warm (avoid drafts in the bathroom) - maintain as pleasant an environment as possible, and provide privacy at all times.

- If available, have a healthcare provider assist the first time.

Unfortunately, accidents can happen quickly in the bathroom try to obtain an emergency response system, which is an electronic device that is usually worn by the elderly to use in case of an emergency. It is usually a pendant or wristband that when pushed will alert the local authorities that help is needed. Contact your local Office on Aging or Police Department for assistance in obtaining a tracking device.

## Mouth Care

A yearly visit to the dentist is essential (some actually make house calls). Electric toothbrushes work well and mouth swabs are available at the pharmacy. Keep lips lubricated to prevent cracking.

## Hair Care

Hairdressers do make house calls. Have dry shampoo available.

## Foot Care

Podiatrists do make house calls - is usually covered by Medicare. Inspect feet daily for open areas and problems.

## Bathroom Assistance

Making adjustments provides more ease and comfort for both the caregiver and the care recipient.

- Have easy access to and nightlights in the bathroom.
- Grab bars (may be covered by Medicare/Medicaid) and a higher toilet seat should be installed.
- Care-recipient should wear easily removable clothing.
- Have available disposable underwear/briefs and wash cloths, a long-neck bottle for rinsing and after-hygiene care flushable wipes.
- Line benches and chairs with vinyl covers. Waterproof pads should be used under bed sheets.
- Purchase incontinent products - adult briefs, pants with snaps and underwear with Velcro, under-patient and incontinent pads and gloves, all of which are washable.
- An open box of baking soda can help relieve odors.

## Medical Supplies and Equipment

Supplies and equipment are costly and always needed. Some of them are covered by Medicare and Medicaid or other health insurance. A reputable medical supply company should know about the extent of what is and is not covered. They may be able to substitute something that is a covered expense. Most suppliers offer free delivery – saves you the trip. Make a note to remind yourself to be sure to get a prescription from your physician.

The following supplies may be needed:

- oxygen
- wheelchairs
- walkers
- hospital beds
- bedside commode (portable toilet)
- under-pads
- diapers/Depends pull-ups
- a cane
- special chairs
- respiratory breathing machine
- nutritional supplements
- Velcro or slip-on shoes
- open-back Velcro or tie night clothes
- snap-close dresses and shirts
- Velcro sweat suits
- other special clothing
- lift chairs, (some lift chairs recline into a bed position).

# Section V

Adult Day Care

Home Health Care Agencies

Assisted Living Facility

Skilled Nursing Home

Continuing Care Retirement Community

Memory Impairment

**Care setting choices have expanded during the past decade. These settings are designed to care for someone who needs custodial care (personal care) with activities of daily living (ADL), which help a person with bathing, eating, dressing, toileting, continence, and transferring.**

Custodial care is less involved than skilled care received at a nursing home. Families who have someone with an illness or disability which requires assistance with activities of daily living, turn to these types of settings for support and caregiver relief.

Payment for these settings are private pay, long-term care insurance, Medicaid and/or sometimes state grants are available.

Visiting your local facilities is one way to find out the cost of care in your neighborhood or use this useful online tool provided by Genworth Insurance Company. A national survey was conducted by CareScout®, April 2016. The survey covers 440 regions and more than 15,000 completed surveys. The user friendly website has an interactive map allowing you to compare not only different types of facility costs but also geographically. https://www.genworth.com/cost-of-care/landing.html

## Adult Day Care

Adult Day Care is an excellent alternative for anyone needing assistance outside the home. This structured health care option provides daily activities that may include bingo, arts and crafts, light exercise instruction, off-site trips, socialization and relief for the caregiver. Most accept memory impairment clients.

Based on an hourly rate, this option is usually less expensive than home care. Funding is sometimes available to those who qualify under different grant programs. Each center's services vary, but most include health monitoring, physical therapy, meals, social activities and transportation. Furthermore, adult day care provides the caregiver with some free time to stay employed and/or relax without having to perform day-to-day care-giving tasks.

Not only the least expensive alternative, adult day care has proven statistics which reduces institutional living 3-5 years, decreases depression, decreases falls, and maintains cognitive functioning for the aging.

## CareScout® Survey

Median annual cost for adult day care based on 5 days per week by 52 weeks.

- Arizona: $21,746
- California: $20,020
- New Jersey: $22,100

Some suggestions to remember:

- Visit more than one center, and spend time observing each center's operation.

- Evaluate the center's staff for competence and levels of compassion.

- Staff-patient ratios are the number of patients assigned to each staff member. These ratios vary by state. They also are different for Adult Day Care Centers than for Nursing Homes or Assisted Living Facilities. Check with your local Department on Aging to find the appropriate ratio for the facility you are evaluating.

- When the opportunity presents itself, talk to some of the other family members who have someone also staying at the center, and ask about their reaction to what they have been experiencing there.

- To possibly help defray some of the costs you are encountering, research the funding that is available through local grants and state funded programs.

## Home Health Care Agencies

Licensed Home Health Care Agencies relieve the caregiver of all background and reference checks for individual caregivers. They should also ensure the caregiver and patient are compatible. They do the work for you. These agencies are bonded which protects you from liability issues. They are also responsible for payroll taxes, social security and disability for their employees.

## CareScout® Survey

Median annual cost for home health care agency based on 44 hours per week by 52 weeks.

- Arizona: $47,979

- California: $54,912

- New Jersey: $50,336

Some suggestions to remember:

- It is very important for there to be compatibility between the caregiver and the care recipient. If the caregiver/worker and care recipient are not compatible do not be afraid to ask the agency to make a change in caregiver assignment.

- Layout specifically your expectations with regard to the extent of care you want, duties to be performed and the hours you will need the caregiver.

- Prior to interviewing the agency, write down some of the needs for care you might want to consider, i.e., light housekeeping, bathing, toileting, laundry and meal preparation.

- Is the worker's appearance neat and clean?

- Obtain agency references and pricing comparisons.

## Assisted Living Facilities

In this setting, a person is somewhat independent and may only require assistance with a few daily living activities. Some of these facilities will have a separate unit for memory impairment patients, and transportation to medical appointments and pleasure trips may sometimes be available. Assistance with dressing and bathing, medication management, personal laundry service and meals are usually included.

Most of these facilities are private, but depending on assets and income in the state where you reside, there could be available financial assistance. So, check with your local Department on Aging and remember it is important to obtain written verification of what will transpire after the resident no longer has the funds needed to pay the facility.

## CareScout® Survey

Median annual cost for assisted living facilities based on 12 months. Private, 1 bedroom.

- Arizona: $42,000
- California: $48,000
- New Jersey: $59,400

Some suggestions to remember:

- Visit one or two of the facilities and spend a day speaking to both the people who are currently residing there, and members of the families.
- Staff-patient ratios are the number of patients assigned to each staff member. These ratios vary by state. They also are different for Assisted Living Facilities than for Nursing Homes or Adult Day Care Centers. Check with your local Department on Aging to find the appropriate ratio for the facility you are evaluating.
- Be sure to thoroughly examine the facility's contract, and make a note of exactly what inclusions and exclusions are included in your monthly payment - some facilities have a la carte fees for certain services.
- Seek the advice of an Elder Law Attorney to review the contract prior to signing.
- Establish at what point the facility will or will not be able to care for the resident.

## Skilled Nursing Home

This kind of facility provides nursing care 24/7, and is regulated by both state and federal guidelines. The setting provides a higher level of personal care, including rehabilitation, nutritional monitoring, various activities, social services and case management. Nursing homes are surveyed annually for clinical and facility competencies. However, it is recommended that you visit the facility at different times and as often as possible to ensure that your family member or other loved one is receiving the best possible care.

## CareScout® Survey

Median annual cost for a skilled nursing home based on 365 days of care.

- Arizona:   Private room $93,075  Semi-private $75,555
- California:   Private room $112,055  Semi-private $91,250
- New Jersey:  Private room $133,835  Semi-private $118,625

Some suggestions to remember:

- Investigate each facility's survey scores - you are entitled to and should do so (check with your local state agencies if necessary).

- Check staff to patient ratio. Staff-patient ratios are the number of patients assigned to each staff member. These ratios vary by state. They also are different for Skilled Nursing Homes than for Adult Day Care Centers or Assisted Living Facilities. Check with your local Department on Aging to find the appropriate ratio for the facility you are evaluating.

## Continuing Care Retirement Communities (CCRC)

Aging in place has evolved into a solution known as Continuing Care Retirement Communities (CCRC). Many people are looking forward to another 40 plus years living independently without having to cook, clean and maintain a home. A CCRC community offers independent living arrangements and if needed in the future, care options at the same location i.e. nursing home, assisted living. This provides a person peace of mind and a place to live for the rest of their lives.

CCRC's costs are not standardized and regulations vary from state to state. There is a non-profit organization called CARF. Founded in 1966 as the Commission on Accreditation of Rehabilitation Facilities, CARF International is an independent, nonprofit accreditor of health and human services. The CARF-CCAC website lists all CCRCs that have been accredited. For more information, go to http://www.carf.org/ccrcListing.aspx.

Another resource is Leading Age, which is an association of 6,000 not-for-profit organizations dedicated to making the United States of America a better place to grow old. For more information go to www.leadingage.org. Here you will find tips on selecting a CCRC.

Some suggestions to remember:

- Oftentimes, there are significant entrance fees.

- Check monthly rental fees and special fees associated with care.

- Review the contracts with an Elder Law Attorney.

- If you are on their waiting list, CCRC's sometimes offer long term care insurance (LTCI).

- Or, the CCRC may require you to buy LTCI which is medically underwritten.

**Memory Impairment**

As a memory impairment disease progresses, there may come a time when professional care is needed. Specialized settings for memory impairment/Alzheimer's may be available such as adult day care or assisted living facilities which will likely have a designated floor for people with dementia. Another option with less of a facility atmosphere are smaller homes designed exclusively for the memory impaired and are located within the community.

Forgetfulness and memory impairment are usually a gradual processes that go unnoticed for some time. When they become noticeable, the person is most likely at the cover-up stage, using the most dominant defense mechanism: denial. The stage that often follows next could include anxiety; when the care recipient experiences a feeling of apprehension, fear, nervousness, or dread accompanied by restlessness or tension. In addition, there is a tendency to be upset and angry at the person who is correcting them (you). The care recipient may tend to withdrawal and avoid being in situations where their inadequacies may surface - simple tasks become difficult, and this makes them angry at themselves.

Some suggestions to remember:

- Try not to challenge or argue with the person.
- Be supportive of their feelings.
- Try not be too impatient.
- Folding laundry is a calming activity.
- Keep the person active.
- Keep things simple.
- Have a current photo on your cell phone.

# Section VI

Do You Need Long Term Care Insurance?

Qualifying for a Long Term Care Insurance Policy

Tax Treatment of Benefits Received

Individual Long Term Care Insurance Policies

Tax Qualified Long Term Care Insurance

Partnership Long Term Care Insurance Policies

Employer Sponsored Long Term Care Insurance Policies

Association Long Term Care Insurance Policies

Federal or State Government Long Term Care Insurance Program

Life Insurance with a Long Term Care Insurance Rider

Annuities

Other Options to Pay for Care

## What you need to know about Long Term Care Insurance and other funding options.

Many insurance carriers (mostly private) issue different types of insurance policies that provide for long term care benefits.(LTCI). These policies typically provide insurance coverage and/or reimbursement for costs incurred when an insured receives care in a nursing facility, assisted living facility, adult day care facility, and even in one's own home. Coverage under these policies typically depends on the type of policy itself, which can vary. Long term care insurance policies may be complex so it is important to try and find the policy that is best for you.

### Do You Need Long Term Care Insurance?

- About 70% of people who reach age 65 are expected to need some form of long-term care at least once in their lifetime. (source AARP)

- Due to illness or accident a person may need hands-on assistance or stand-by assistance which is often referred to as Personal Care or Custodial Care.

- 59% of Caregivers reported "less stress" was a side benefit of their loved one owning LTCI. (Genworth Beyond Dollars Study)

- If you have a low monthly income or assets, then you probably do not need this policy because you would likely be eligible for government assistance. (Section III Medicaid)

- If you have a high income and a large number of assets, then you may choose to self-insure or buy lower LTCI benefits to supplement income/assets.

- You want to avoid dependence on spouse, children and/or government programs.

- Make sure you will be able to afford premiums over a long period of time.

- Keep the premium affordable in case the premium increases.

- Having a policy will give you more choices as to where you will receive care.

- Worksheets are available in Section VIII.

### Qualifying for a Long Term Care Insurance Policy

- Insurance companies will look at your medical history when you apply for coverage.

- Policies are medically underwritten. Once you have a diagnosis, it may be harder to qualify for a policy. Accurately answer all questions on the application. Shop around and try to "pre-qualify" before submitting an application. Because once declined from one insurance company that information is available to all companies. Underwriting practices will be different from company to company.

- Medically underwritten at time of application is the best option in order to avoid the insurance company denying benefits when you need them. Underwriting is important because people would not buy a policy until they needed it.

- If you purchase a policy prior to developing one of the conditions listed below, then your policy will cover the care you need for that condition.

Disqualifying factors could include but not limited to:

- Already in need of help with Activities of Daily Living (ADL's)
- Been diagnosed with Alzheimer's or any form of Dementia
- Have AIDS or AIDS-related complex (ARC)
- Have progressive neurological condition such as Parkinson's Disease or Multiple Sclerosis
- Stroke within the past two years or history of strokes
- Metastatic Cancer.

## Tax Treatment of Benefits Received

**Expense incurred method**: Once there's an expense for an eligible service, the insurer pays benefits either to you or your provider. The coverage pays either the amount of the expense or your policy's dollar limit, whichever is less. Most policies sold today use the expense-incurred method. Benefits from reimbursement policies, which pay for the actual services a beneficiary receives, are not included in income.

**Indemnity or disability**: Method of paying benefits where the benefit is a set dollar amount that isn't based on the specific service received or the expenses incurred. Once the company decides you're eligible for benefits because you're receiving eligible long term care services, it pays the set amount up to the limit of the policy. Benefits from per diem or indemnity policies, which pay a predetermined amount each day, are not included in income except amounts that exceed the beneficiary's total qualified long-term care expenses or $340 per day (in 2016), whichever is greater.

## Types of Long Term Care Insurance Policies Available

## Individual Long Term Care Insurance Policies

Nursing home only policies were introduced in the 1980's and now there are many more choices available.

- LTCI Policies are not standardized.
- Some policies may only cover Certified Nursing Home Facilities.
- Some policies may only cover licensed Home Health Care.
- Comprehensive policies may cover Nursing Home, Home Health Care, Adult Day Care, Respite Care, Hospice Care, Caregiver Training, Home Modifications, and Chore Services.
- State-licensed facilities are usually a requirement for benefits.
- Joint policies can cover more than one person and are commonly called "shared care".

- Care Management services help with evaluation of need and work with family to develop a plan of care.

- Most LTCI policies require a doctor to certify the illness will last 90 days or more. Example - A hip replacement will not qualify as a claim because the insured is expected to recover and be walking within 90 days or less.

- Discounts applied towards premium might be offered to spouses applying together, siblings, civil unions, and/or people who live together for a certain number of years.

## Tax-Qualified Long Term Care Insurance

- HIPPA (1996) created "Tax-Qualified" LTCI policies. These policies offer tax deductions and consumer protections.

- Grandfather rules apply to policies bought prior to January 1, 1997.

- HIPPA standards:
    > Guaranteed renewable.
    > Chronically ill: unable to perform at least two activities of daily living (ADL) without substantial assistance from another person for at least 90 days. Or, if you have a cognitive impairment and need substantial supervision to protect your safety and health.
    > Follow plan of care prescribed by a licensed health care practitioner.

- Itemized tax deduction: medical expenses includes a portion of LTCI premiums.

- Age based maximum deduction of premiums are taken if expenses for unreimbursed medical expenses (including Medicare premiums) are greater than 10% of adjusted gross income. (consult your tax advisor)

- Business owners/corporations have different options.

- For individuals, there is a maximum deduction of LTCI premium set by the IRS, any amount above the limit is not considered to be a medical expense.

## 2017 Chart Long Term Care Insurance Annual Premium

| Attained age before end of tax year | Maximum deduction for tax year |
|---|---|
| 40 or younger | $410 |
| 40 to 50 | $770 |
| 50 to 60 | $1,530 |
| 60 to 70 | $4,090 |
| Older than 70 | $5,110 |

## Partnership Long Term Care Insurance Policies

A partnership between the insured who is a resident of a state which chooses to participate in Partnership program and the insured purchases a LTCI partnership plan within that state to help reduce Medicaid expenses.

- Must be federally tax-qualified plans and include certain consumer protections. Offered in most states.
- Must include inflation rider for all persons younger than age 75.
- Must have compound inflation for persons younger than age 61.
- Some level of inflation for all persons' ages 61 to 75.
- Designed to help manage the impact of spending down for Medicaid.
- In most states you can qualify for Medicaid and keep income and assets equal to the amount of claims your partnership policy paid.
- If you move your residence, most states will reciprocate the agreement.

## Employer Sponsored Long Term Care Insurance

- HIPPA gave employers a federal tax benefit when they pay their employees premiums.
- Owners and key employees can have their own benefits.
- Most "Group" policies are voluntary enrollment and paid for by the employee.
- Group discounts could apply.
- Convenient payroll deduction.
- Medical questions may be less stringent than applying for an individual policy.
- Group premium rates could be offered to spouses and other relatives of the employee. However, a more stringent medical questionnaire may apply.
- The "Group" coverage is usually portable, meaning if you leave that company your coverage may continue and billed to you directly.

## Association Long Term Care Insurance Policies

- Usually an additional premium discount is applied for members.
- Medically underwritten.
- Members design their own policy benefits.
- Some restrictions may apply, regarding how long you have to be and/or stay a member of the association.
- Check portability if you no longer belong to the association.

## Federal or State Government Long Term Care Insurance Program

- Premiums are not paid by the Federal Government.
- Insurance coverage is underwritten by insurance companies.
- Compare premiums and benefits with other policies sold by insurance carriers.

## Life Insurance with a Long Term Care Insurance Rider (life/long-term care)

- A percentage of the death benefit is used while you are alive for long term care expenses.
- The percentage will be paid out daily or monthly.
- Percentages will vary from carriers. Example: $200,000 death benefit times 2% of death benefit would provide $4,000 monthly benefit towards care. Or, a 3% of death benefit option would provide $6,000 monthly benefit towards care.
- The death benefit will be reduced by the amount used for care.
- Whole life contracts will not have future premium increases.
- Death benefit is guaranteed to go to the named beneficiary less money paid out towards care.
- Policies accumulate cash value.
- LTCI benefit could be a rider with an additional premium.
- Tax qualified life insurance with long term care benefits must meet the same federal standards as tax qualified LTCI policies.
- Shop around and compare.

## Annuities

- Can create an income stream to pay for care.
- Some annuity contracts will continue the monthly income even after the principle investment has been exhausted.
- IRA money can be used.
- Non-Qualified money can be used.
- Savings can be used.
- Shop around and compare.

## Other Options to Pay for Care

- Current cash value within a life insurance policy.
- Reverse mortgage.
- 1035 exchange is a provision in the tax code which allows you, as a policyholder, to transfer funds from a life insurance, endowment or annuity to a new policy, without having to pay taxes.

# Section VII

How Much Will a Long Term Care Insurance Plan Pay?

Long Term Care Insurance Claim

Eligibility for Benefits

Optional Long Term Care Insurance Riders

**All long term care insurance policies have similar "options" that were available to the insured when the insured decided to purchase coverage.**

The insured might not remember everything about their policy but they may remember if they have a "Limit" on benefits available. This is referred to as "Lifetime Benefit" or "Policy Limit/Pool of Money" The insured's insurance carrier will be able to provide specific information. A common fear among policy holders is the fear of running out of coverage.

This is how it works:

- At the time of application, the insured decided how much "Daily or Monthly" benefit they want. This is called the "maximum daily/monthly benefit".

- The insured decided how long they wanted the insurance. company to pay out the benefits in terms of years. Or, selected a benefit "Policy Limit/Pool". This is called the "Lifetime Benefit."

- Therefore, the "Lifetime Benefit" or "Policy Limit" is a multiple of Daily Benefit times the Benefit Period.

For example:

Daily Benefit is $100 per day and Benefit Period is 3 years (1095 days)
$100 x 1095 days = $109,500 in Lifetime Benefit

Another example:

Monthly Benefit is $4,500 per month and Benefit Period is 6 years (72 months)
$4,500 x 72 months = $324,000 in Lifetime Benefit

The Elimination Period (deductible) will need to be satisfied before benefits begin.

## Long Term Care Insurance Claim

The industry uses the term "benefit triggers" to describe when an insured maybe considered "Eligible for Benefits." If the insured is unable to perform a certain number of Activities of Daily Living (ADL) or, most policies will pay benefit for cognitive impairment (Alzheimer's disease or other form of dementia).

**Activities of Daily Living (ADL)**: Typically, a policy pays benefits when the insured can't do a certain number of the ADL, such as two of the six or three of the six.

1. Bathing: Washing oneself in either a tub or shower. This activity includes getting in or out of the tub or shower.

2. Continence: Being able to control bowel and bladder function or, if you can't, being able to manage needed personal hygiene (such as catheter or colostomy bag).

3. Dressing: Putting on and taking off all items of clothing and any necessary braces, fasteners, or artificial limbs.

4. Eating: Feeding yourself by getting food into the body from a receptacle (such as a plate, cup, or table).

5. Toileting: Getting to and from the toilet, getting on and off the toilet, and doing related personal hygiene.

6. Transferring: Moving into and out of a bed, chair, or wheelchair.

Or, Cognitive Impairment:

- A loss of short or long term memory; difficulty knowing people, places, or the time or season; loss of the ability to make good decisions; or loss of safety awareness.

- Alzheimer's disease or other form of dementia.

Most Exclusions are:

- Mental or nervous disorder or disease, other than Alzheimer's disease or dementia.

- Alcohol or drug addiction.

- Illness or injury caused by an act of war.

- Treatment in a government facility or that government has already paid for.

- Attempted suicide or intentionally self-inflicted injuries.

**Eligibility for Benefits**

Contracts will vary in coverage - Most policies require a Doctor (the insureds) to certify the illness will last 90 days or more. Example - A hip replacement will not qualify as a claim because the insured is expected to recover and be walking within 90 days or less.

**Elimination Period (EP) (sometimes called the deductible or waiting period)**

It is the insureds responsibility to satisfy the amount of days specified within their policy with Qualified Long Term Care prior to the insurance company paying the daily/monthly benefit. The elimination period can be 0,20,30,60, 90 or 100 days. The elimination Period is defined within the policy:

- Satisfied once in your lifetime?

- Episode of Care?

- Non-consecutive days?

- Consecutive days?

- Separate elimination period for different levels of care?

- What type of services can be applied to satisfy the EP?

# Calculation of Days towards Satisfying the Elimination Period (EP)

- Calendar Days: you may not need care every day of the week. However, this method will credit a full 7 days towards the EP, even if you are not receiving care on those days.

- Service Days: only qualified days which you are receiving care will count towards the EP.

*Check the policy and or the outline of coverage for specific details.*

## Optional Riders - Inflation Protection/Benefit Increase

The cost of nursing home care has increased around 7% every year. (Prudential Long Term Care Cost Study 2010)

- $150 a day in 2016 will cost $398 a day in 20 years.

- Inflation protection rider will automatically increase your daily/monthly and lifetime benefit.

- Premium cost will increase between 25% to 40%.

Rider Options

- **Automatic Increases**: fixed percentage increase every year or for a predetermined period of years 10 or 20.

- **Compound rate** is more expensive because the dollar amount added will increase every year.

- **Simple rate** will add the same dollar amount every year.

- **Special offer or Non-Automatic Inflation** every so many years the insured will receive a letter to increase the daily/monthly benefit. Usually offered with no medical questions, additional benefit will require additional premium calculated based on attained age.

| Rate of Inflation | 2015 | 2020 | 2025 | 2030 | 2035 |
|---|---|---|---|---|---|
| *LTCI Daily Benefit Starting at $200 per day.* | | | | | |
| Compounding 5% | $200 | $255 | $326 | $416 | $531 |
| Simple 5% | $200 | $250 | $300 | $350 | $400 |

## Non-Forfeiture Benefit Rider

- Premium cost will increase 10% - 100%

- Amount of premium paid and for how long will determine the level of benefits.

- Reduced paid-up - same benefit period but with a lower daily benefit.

- Shortened benefit period - same daily benefit with a reduced benefit period.

- Extended Term - must use coverage within a certain period of time.

- Return of Premium - all or part of premiums are returned.

## Contingent Non-Forfeiture Benefits

This is usually built in (varies by states) and offers a way to keep your policy if the insurance company has increased the premium (based on a table of increases).

- Reduce benefits of current policy so the premium will remain the same.
- Paid-up policy would shorten the benefit period with no future premiums due.
- Keep the same benefits and pay the higher premium.

## Waiver of Premium Rider

Once the claims department has determined you are eligible for benefits and they are paying out claim, the insurance company will no longer require the insured to pay the premium. This could be effective right away or after 60 or 90 days, depending on the policy.

## Restoration of Benefits Rider

- Insured qualified for a claim and used some of the "Lifetime Benefit" and did not exhaust the policy benefits.
- 180 consecutive days goes by and the insured remains ineligible for benefits, the amount of benefit used will be restored to the "Lifetime Benefit".

## Premium Refund at Death Rider

- Total dollar amount of premiums paid minus any claims.
- Return of premium if death occurs prior to a certain age i.e. 65 or 75.
- Return of premium at death.

# Section VIII

Cost of Care Worksheet

What's Your Plan Worksheet

Exploring Long Term Care Insurance Worksheet

# Cost of Care Worksheet

After exploring and evaluating the cost of care in your area and knowing the amount of income/assets you have you will be able to determine how much per month you will need for care in an adult day care, home care or nursing facility. Remember, this is in addition to your current living expenses and if you take a distribution from an IRA/pension it will be taxed as ordinary income.

Visiting your local facilities is one way to find out the cost of care in your neighborhood or use this useful online tool provided by Genworth Insurance Company. The national survey was conducted by CareScout®, April 2016. The survey covers 440 regions and over 15,000 completed surveys. The user friendly website has an interactive map allowing you to compare not only different types of facility costs but also geographically. https://www.genworth.com/cost-of-care/landing.html

## A. Cost of care where you live now.

Monthly cost of care: ______________________________________

Adult Day $________________________    Home Health Care $________________________

Assisted Living $________________________    Nursing Home $________________________

## B. Cost of care if you plan on moving closer to children.

Monthly cost of care: ______________________________________

Adult Day $________________________    Home Health Care $________________________

Assisted Living $________________________    Nursing Home $________________________

## C. Cost of care if you plan on retiring to a different state.

Monthly cost of care: ______________________________________

Adult Day $________________________    Home Health Care $________________________

Assisted Living $________________________    Nursing Home $________________________

# What's Your Plan Worksheet

Planning to die early, is not a plan.

Long term care insurance policies and planning techniques (life insurance with LTCI rider and/or Annuities) can seem overwhelming, keep it simple and answer the questions below. Circumstances vary from peron to person so there are not any "correct" answers.

If the event occurred, the loss of two activities of daily living or severe cognitive impairment (Alzheimer's/Dementia) and a medical professional has determined the illness will last 90 days or more. Ask yourself:

How much will it cost and how much additional money per month do you need to cover all or part of the cost of care?

Will your spouse be healthy enough to be able to care for you?      Yes   No

Will your spouse have the time to be able to care for you or will they still be working?

Will your children be healthy enough to be able to care for you?      Yes   No

Will your children have the time to be able to care for you or will they still be working?

Would you prefer to stay in your home or go to a care facility?

Will you stay home with family and visit Adult Day Care to ease your caregiver's schedule?

Are your income and assets low enough to apply for Medicaid?      Yes   No

Are you a Veteran?      Yes   No

Do you have enough income and assets to consider living within a Continuing Care Retirement Community (CCRC)?

Are you healthy enough to obtain a medically underwritten LTCI policy?      Yes   No

Starting today, let's work together. Lorraine has specialized in long term care insurance planning since 1997. Technology has brought us all closer together therefore, no matter where you live in the United States, we can work together on this extremely important matter.

To be efficient and understand you and your family better, complete the information below. One of the most important parts of planning is having the right coverage for you, before you need it. You can download the forms in this section from my website at KeySolutionsForCaregivers.com to complete and email to LorraineSpiotta@gmail.com for a no-obligation Long Term Care Insurance consultation. Lorraine is not affiliated with any government agency. By responding and submitting requested materials, you may be contacted by an insurance agent.

## Step 1: Start with these "base" selections

| | | | | | |
|---|---|---|---|---|---|
| Monthly benefit | $2,000 | $3,000 | $4,500 | $6,000 | $8,000 |
| Benefit period | 2 years | 3 years | 4 years | 5 years | 6 years | 10 years |
| Elimination period | 0 | 30 | 60 | 90 | 100 |
| Inflation rider | Compound | Simple |
| Premium discount | Spousal | Civil union | Sibling | Association |
| Premium payment option | Annual | Semi-annual | Quarterly | Monthly | Lump sum |

## Step 2:  Who are you?

Your name: _______________________     Spouse/Partner: _______________________

Address: _______________________

City: _______________________     State: _______________     Zip code: _______________

Phone: _______________________     Email: _______________________

How many children/ages: _______________________

Your date of birth: ____________     Height: ____________     Weight: ____________     Smoker: ____________

Spouse/Partner date of birth: ____________     Height: ____________     Weight: ____________     Smoker: ____________

List all prescription drugs: _______________________________________________

_______________________________________________________________________

_______________________________________________________________________

_______________________________________________________________________

Medical diagnosis, operations and/or hospitalizations within the past 10 years: _______

_______________________________________________________________________

_______________________________________________________________________

_______________________________________________________________________

## Income

Salary: _________________________ Social Security: _____________________

Pension: ________________________ IRA: ______________________________

Other: __________________________

## Assets

Home value: _____________________ Mortgage balance: ____________________

Other home value: ________________ CD/Money market: _____________________

Checking: _______________________ Savings: ____________________________

Annuity (non qualified): ___________ Annuity (qualified): ___________________

Type of life insurance:            Term            Universal            Whole life

Life insurance death benefit: _________________________________________

Life insurance cash value: ___________________________________________

Investments: _____________________________________________________

Investments: _____________________________________________________

Other: _________________________________________________________

# Section IX

Resources

Parting Thoughts

About the Authors

# Resource Websites and Phone Numbers

**Aging Life Care Association**
www.aginglifecare.org                    N/A

**Alzheimer's Association**
www.alz.org                              (800) 272-3900

**American Academy of Home Care Medicine**
www.aahcm.org                            (847) 375-4719

**American Health Care Association**
www.ahcancal.org                         N/A

**Commission on Accreditation of Rehabilitation Facilities**
www.carf.org                             (888) 281-6531

**Eldercare Locator**
www.eldercare.gov                        (800) 677-1116

**Leading Age**
www.leadingage.org                       (202) 783-2242

**National Academy of Elder Law Attorneys**
www.naela.org                            N/A

**US Department of Health & Human Services Administration on Aging**
www.aoa.gov                              N/A

**US Department of Housing & Urban Development (HUD)**
www.hud.gov                              (202) 708-1112

# Emergency                911

For help when buying a Medigap policy or long-term care insurance contact your state SHIP (State Health Insurance Assistance Program). State contact information can be found via www.shiptacenter.org.

The websites and phone numbers listed on this page were correct at the time of printing. Sometimes agency information changes.

Finally, and to some degree maybe most importantly, if you are the primary caregiver understand that caregiving responsibilities can and will sometimes be overwhelming and you need to:

- ☐ Make a plan of care so it is easy for others to help.

- ☐ Work toward a positive relationship with the care recipient and others who are helping you to provide that care.

- ☐ Delegate – one person can't handle everything (not even you!).

- ☐ Use this handbook to your advantage and make whatever journal entries you want to about your feeling, impressions or anything else that comes up.

- ☐ Communicate with family and friends, and be sure to take a break; go out to lunch, read a book, have a quiet day for yourself.

- ☐ Consider light exercise or yoga to clear your mind.

- ☐ Find a support group for yourself.

- ☐ Self-care is not selfish! If you are worn down and become ill, who will provide care? Have a plan for continual self-care and a back-up plan for unexpected events that could affect caregiving.

# About the Authors

## Lorraine Kenney Spiotta, CLU, ChFC

Since 1997, Lorraine has worked to bring long term care insurance policies and a "peace of mind" to a diverse group of clients. The President and founder of Senior Long-Term Care Insurance Brokerage, Inc., Lorraine successfully completed the advance training and educational requirements for the prestigious Charter Life Underwriter (CLU) and Chartered Financial Consultant (ChFC).

Widely recognized and acknowledged in New Jersey as one of the foremost spokespersons in the Long-Term Care Insurance industry, Lorraine is the author of an article which appeared in Assisted Living Success Magazine entitled *A Call for Partnership Between Long-Term Care Insurance and You*. With her expertise in human resource issues related to elder care, she served as a Commissioner on the New Jersey Commission on Aging. Contact Lorraine at (732) 651-1495 or LorraineSpiotta@gmail.com.

## Tracey Christenson Wolfman, RN, BSN, MA

Tracey is a Registered Nurse and owner of We Care Adult Care, Inc. in Middletown, NJ. With more than 30 years of experience working with seniors and their caregivers in the areas of long-term care, hospital care, assisted living, home care and adult day care, she holds a BSN Degree from Monmouth University and a Master's degree in Nursing Administration from Columbia University.

As the number one Adult Day Care Center in Monmouth County, Tracey's company won the 2003 Small Business Leadership Award. Throughout New Jersey, and as a mentor and inspiration for other nurses who want to become entrepreneurs, she is a recognized speaker on Adult Day Care and senior issues. Tracey is also an expert on helping seniors and cargivers find caregiving services that will more than adequately fulfill both their needs. Contact Tracey at (732) 741-7363 or www.wecareadultcare.com.

# Section X

Caregive Journal and Notes

# Caregiver Journal and Notes

# Caregiver Journal and Notes

# Caregiver Journal and Notes

# Caregiver Journal and Notes

# Caregiver Journal and Notes

# Caregiver Journal and Notes

# Caregiver Journal and Notes

# Caregiver Journal and Notes

# Caregiver Journal and Notes

# Caregiver Journal and Notes

# Caregiver Journal and Notes

# Caregiver Journal and Notes

# Caregiver Journal and Notes

# Caregiver Journal and Notes

# Caregiver Journal and Notes

# Caregiver Journal and Notes

# Caregiver Journal and Notes

# Caregiver Journal and Notes

# Caregiver Journal and Notes

# Caregiver Journal and Notes

# Caregiver Journal and Notes

# Caregiver Journal and Notes

# Caregiver Journal and Notes

# Caregiver Journal and Notes

# Caregiver Journal and Notes

# Caregiver Journal and Notes

# Caregiver Journal and Notes

# Does your business serve the aging population and their families?

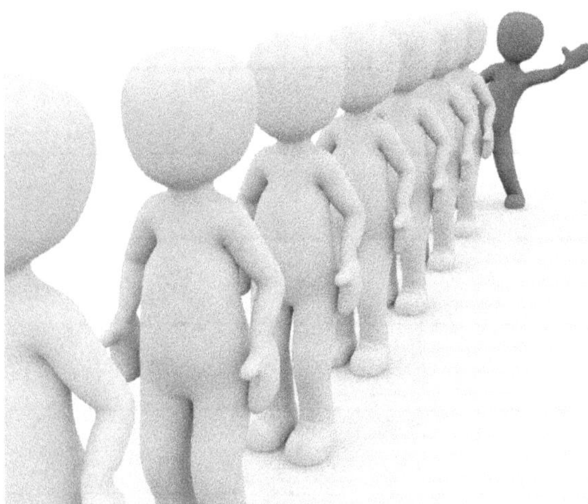

Why waste marketing dollars on water bottles, key chains, refrigerator magnets, print and/or social media?

Stand out from the crowd and personalize this book with your logo and company information. Your contact information is invaluable and so is the information within *Key Solutions for Caregivers.*

**Contact keysolutionsfor@gmail.com for the best marketing tool on the market today!**

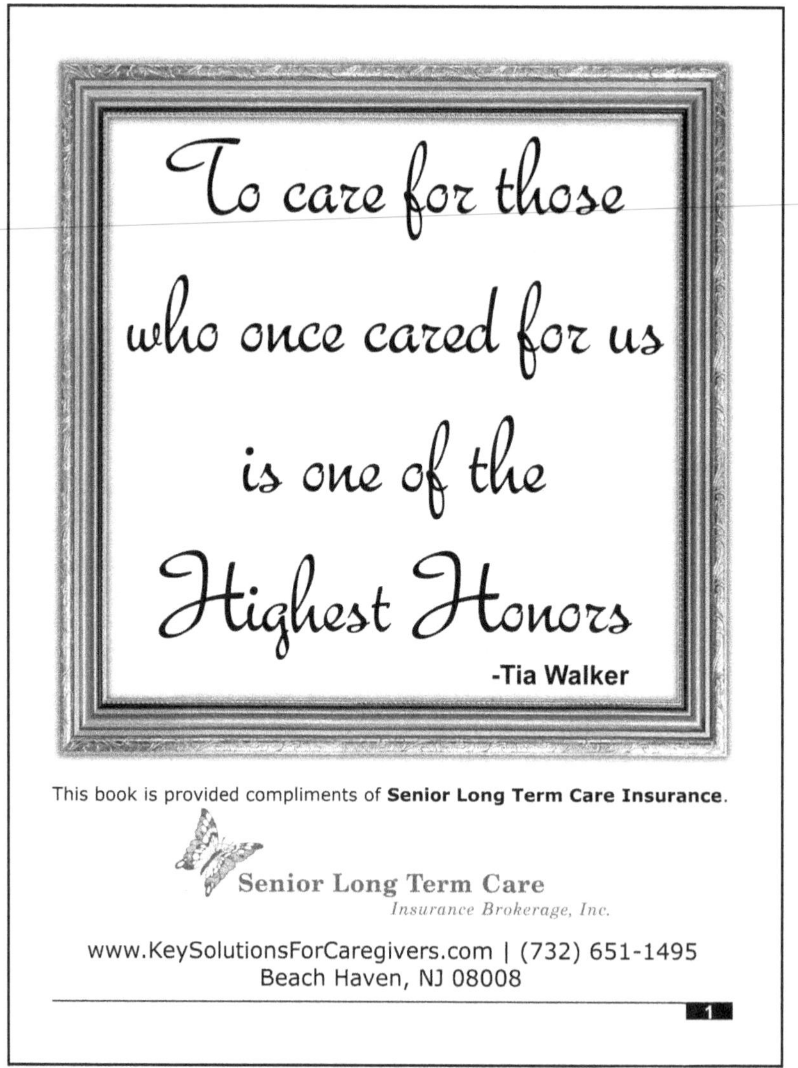

# Want to be an author?

I am on a nationwide search for co-authors who have an expertise related to planning and guidance for the aging population and their families such as; elder law, financial planning, Alzheimer's, Parkinson's, cancer, home health care agencies, concierge physicians, etcetera.

If you or someone you know wants to be an author, has little time to complete an entire book on their own, wants to stand out as an expert within their field and has a willingness to collaborate,  there might be a spot available in the Key Solutions series.

The next books in the Key Solutions for... series will include chapters from *Key Solutions for Caregivers* and will add a twist into the direction of the co-author's expertise.

*Key Solutions for Caregivers* is the first of the series. This book provides a place to record important personal information which needs to be available for hospitalizations and financial assistant programs. It also includes specific information regarding care setting choices, tips for the caregiver in various situations and information about Medicare, Medicaid and long term care insurance.

If you or someone you know has an idea and expertise for the next Key Solution for... series, contact keysolutionsfor@gmail.com.

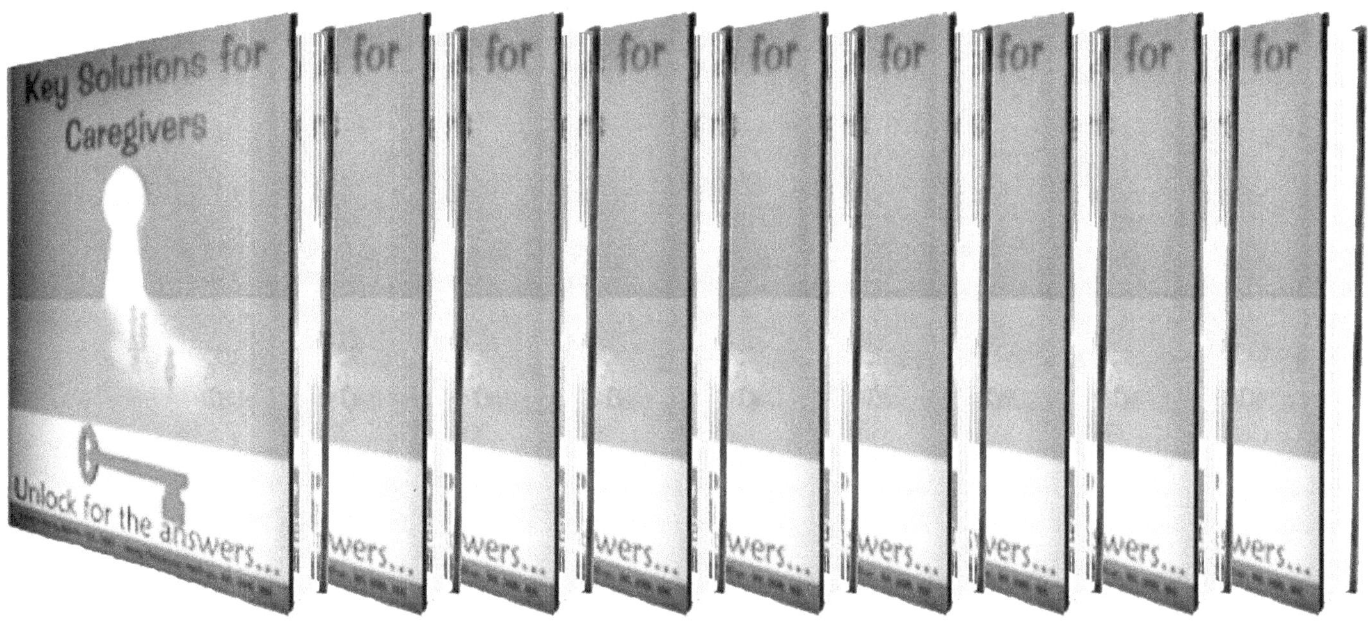